Copyright ©2020 SHARON MCQUEEN All rights reserved.

No part of this publication may be reproduced, distributed, or transmitted in any form or by any means, including photocopying, recording, or other electronic or mechanical methods, without the prior written permission of the publisher, except in the case of brief quotations embodied in the critical reviews and certain other noncommercial uses permitted by the copyright law.

Table of Contents

Introduction

Around 300 BCE, a surgeon in ancient Greece named Herophilus became the first person to formally describe the pancreas as a gland. However, the organ didn't get its name until about 400 years later, when another Greek surgeon and anatomist named Ruphos dubbed it the pankreas, meaning "all flesh"—possibly because of its lack of bone or cartilage. (The plural of pancreas, by the way, is pancreata or pancreases.) Later, in the 16th century, people started referring to a dish of cooked calf or lamb pancreas as "sweetbreads." That name possibly stems from bræd, the Old English word for "flesh."

Pancreatitis is pathologic inflammation of the pancreas. Your pancreas sits behind your stomach, near your small intestine. It releases enzymes that help you digest food and also regulates how your body manages glucose.

Pancreatitis is inflammation of the pancreas. The pancreas is a large gland behind the stomach, close to the first part of the small intestine, called the duodenum. The pancreas has two main functions—to make insulin and to make digestive juices, or enzymes, to help you digest food. These enzymes digest food in the intestine. Pancreatitis occurs when the enzymes damage the pancreas, which causes inflammation. Pancreatitis can be acute or chronic. Either form is serious and can lead to complications.

You could live without your pancreas, but it wouldn't be easy. For one, you would need to give yourself insulin shots on a daily basis because you would develop diabetes. A helping of enzyme pills would also be needed to help you digest food. It's clear that the 6-inch-long pancreas, located behind your stomach, has crucial functions—and that's why diseases like pancreatic cancer and pancreatitis are often so devastating.

Pancreatitis can come and go quickly, or it can be a chronic problem. Treatment will depend on whether your pancreatitis is acute or chronic.

What is Pancreatitis?
Pancreatitis is a disease in which your pancreas becomes inflamed.

The pancreas is a large gland behind your stomach and next to your small intestine. Your pancreas does two main things:

- It releases powerful digestive enzymes into your small intestine to help you digest food.

- It releases insulin and glucagon into your bloodstream. These hormones help your body control how it uses food for energy.

Your pancreas can be damaged when digestive enzymes begin working before your pancreas releases them.

Types of Pancreatitis

The two forms of pancreatitis are acute and chronic.

Acute pancreatitis is sudden inflammation that lasts a short time. It can range from mild discomfort to a severe, life-threatening illness. Most people with acute pancreatitis recover completely after getting the right treatment. In severe cases, acute pancreatitis can cause bleeding, serious tissue damage, infection, and cysts. Severe pancreatitis can also harm other vital organs such as the heart, lungs, and kidneys.

Acute pancreatitis is a main cause of hospital admissions for gastrointestinal issues. According to the National Institute of Diabetes and Digestive and Kidney Diseases (NIDDK), around 275,000 Americans are admitted to the hospital for acute pancreatitis every year.

The onset of acute pancreatitis is often very sudden. The inflammation usually clears up within several days after treatment begins, but some cases could require a hospital stay.

Acute pancreatitis is much more common in adults than in children. Gallstones are the primary cause of acute pancreatitis in adults.

The condition can also develop into chronic pancreatitis, especially if you smoke or regularly drink alcohol.

Chronic pancreatitis is long-lasting inflammation. It most often happens after an episode of acute pancreatitis. Another top cause is drinking lots of alcohol for a long period of time. Damage to your pancreas from heavy alcohol use may not cause symptoms for many years, but then you may suddenly have severe pancreatitis symptoms.

Chronic pancreatitis is an inflammation of the pancreas that comes back consistently or occurs over a long period of time.

People with chronic pancreatitis can have permanent damage to their pancreas and other complications. Scar tissue develops from this continuing inflammation.

Pancreatitis can damage cells that produce insulin, a hormone released by the pancreas that regulates the amount of sugar in your blood. This leads to diabetes in about 45 percent of people with chronic pancreatitis.

Long-term alcohol use causes around 70 percent of cases of chronic pancreatitis in adults. Autoimmune and genetic diseases, such as cystic fibrosis, can also cause chronic pancreatitis in some people.

Necrotizing pancreatitis

Severe cases of acute pancreatitis can develop into necrotizing pancreatitis, which refers to the death of cells due to disease. This occurs in about 10 percentTrusted Source of acute pancreatitis cases, typically when pancreatitis is left untreated.

Inflammation from pancreatitis can cause digestive enzymes to leak into the pancreas. This can result in damage and death of the tissue, leading to necrotizing pancreatitis. Your doctor may order an abdominal ultrasound or CT scan to diagnose the condition.

If you have necrotizing pancreatitis, your doctor may take a sample of the dead tissue to make sure it hasn't become infected. If you have an infection, you'll likely need to take antibiotics and may need to have the dead tissue removed.

The infection of dead tissue increases the risk of death from necrotizing pancreatitis, so it's very important to seek treatment as quickly as possible.

Pancreatitis Symptoms
Symptoms of acute pancreatitis:

- Fever

- Higher heart rate

- Nausea and vomiting

- Swollen and tender belly

- Pain in the upper part of your belly that goes into your back. Eating may make it worse, especially foods high in fat.

Symptoms of chronic pancreatitis
The symptoms of chronic pancreatitis are similar to those of acute pancreatitis. But you may also have:

- Constant pain in your upper belly that radiates to your back. This pain may be disabling.

- Diarrhea and weight loss because your pancreas isn't releasing enough enzymes to break down food

- Upset stomach and vomiting

- Pancreatitis Causes and Risk Factors

Acute pancreatitis causes include:

- Autoimmune diseases

- Drinking lots of alcohol

- Infections

- Gallstones

- Medications

- Metabolic disorders

- Surgery

- Trauma

In up to 15% of people with acute pancreatitis, the

cause is unknown.

Chronic pancreatitis causes include:

- Cystic fibrosis
- Family history of pancreas disorders
- Gallstones
- High triglycerides
- Longtime alcohol use

Medications
In about 20% to 30% of cases, the cause of chronic pancreatitis is unknown. People with chronic pancreatitis are usually men between ages 30 and 40.

Pancreatitis Complications
Pancreatitis can have severe complications, including:

- Diabetes if there's damage to the cells that produce insulin
- Infection of your pancreas

- Kidney failure

Malnutrition if your body can't get enough nutrients from the food you eat because of a lack of digestive enzymes

Pancreatic cancer
Pancreatic necrosis, when tissues die because your pancreas isn't getting enough blood

Problems with your breathing when chemical changes in your body affect your lungs

Pseudocysts, when fluid collects in pockets on your pancreas. They can burst and become infected.

Pancreatitis Diagnosis
To diagnose acute pancreatitis, your doctor tests your blood to measure two digestive enzymes: amylase and lipase. High levels of these two enzymes mean you probably have acute pancreatitis.

Your doctor will likely use a combination of blood tests and imaging studies to make a diagnosis. If you have acute pancreatitis, you'll have severe abdominal pain and blood tests may show a significant rise in your level of pancreatic enzymes.

Different types of ultrasound, MRI, and CT scans can reveal the anatomy of your pancreas, signs of inflammation, and information about the biliary and pancreatic ducts. A fecal fat test can also determine if your stools have fat content that's higher than normal.

Other tests can include:

- Pancreatic function test to find out whether your pancreas is making the right amounts of digestive enzymes

- Ultrasound, CT scan, and MRI, which make images of your pancreas

- ERCP, in which your doctor uses a long tube with a camera on the end to look at your pancreatic and bile ducts

- Biopsy, in which your doctor uses a needle to remove a small piece of tissue from your pancreas to be studied

In some cases, your doctor may test your blood and poop to confirm the diagnosis. They may also do a glucose tolerance test to measure damage to the cells in your pancreas that make insulin.

Pancreatitis Treatment

Treatment for acute pancreatitis

You'll probably need to stay in the hospital, where your treatment may include:

- Antibiotics if your pancreas is infected

- Intravenous (IV) fluids, given through a needle

- Low-fat diet or fasting. You might need to stop eating so your pancreas can recover. In this case, you'll get nutrition through a feeding tube.

- Pain medicine

- If your case is more severe, your treatment might include:

- ERCP to take out gallstones if they're blocking your bile or pancreatic ducts

- Gallbladder surgery if gallstones caused your pancreatitis

- Pancreas surgery to clean out fluid or dead or diseased tissue

Pancreatic function test

The pancreatic function test, also called the secretin stimulation test, shows whether your pancreas is responding normally to secretin. Secretin is a hormone that causes your pancreas to release a fluid that helps digest food.

During the test, your doctor will run a tube through your nose or throat and down into your small intestine. They'll inject secretin into your vein, then take samples of fluid through the tube.

Your doctor will send the fluid to a lab to help diagnose pancreatitis or other conditions affecting your pancreas.

Treatment for chronic pancreatitis

If you have chronic pancreatitis, you might need more treatments, including:

- Insulin to treat diabetes

- Pain medicine

- Pancreatic enzymes to help your body get enough nutrients from your food

- Surgery or procedures to relieve pain, help with drainage, or treat blockages

Pancreatitis Prevention

Because many cases of pancreatitis are caused by alcohol abuse, prevention often focuses on limiting how much you drink or not drinking at all. If your drinking is a concern, talk to your doctor or health care professional about an alcohol treatment center. A support group such as Alcoholics Anonymous could also help.

Stop smoking, follow your doctor's and dietitian's advice about your diet, and take your medications so you'll have fewer and milder attacks of pancreatitis.

Pancreatitis diet

A low-fat, healthy diet plays a major role in recovering from pancreatitis. People with chronic pancreatitis in particular need to be careful about the amount of fat they consume, since their pancreas function has become compromised. Try to limit or avoid the following foods:

- red meat

- fried food

- full-fat dairy

- sugary desserts

- sweetened beverages

- caffeine

- alcohol

Eat small meals throughout the day to put less stress on your digestive system. Stick to foods that are high in protein and antioxidants, and drink lots of fluids to stay hydrated.

Your doctor might also give you vitamin supplements to ensure that you're getting the nutrients you need.

Pancreatitis home remedies

It's important to see your doctor if you think you have pancreatitis, especially if you have consistent pain in your abdomen. There are steps you can take at home to supplement your treatment and help prevent pancreatitis.

Lifestyle changes

Stop smoking tobacco and curb drinking alcohol in excess to help you heal more quickly and completely. Discuss these issues with your doctor if you need help.

Maintaining a healthy weight can help you avoid gallstones, a primary cause of pancreatitis. Eating a balanced diet and staying hydrated can also help you recover from and prevent pancreatitis.

Alternative techniques for pain control

You'll probably be given IV pain medication in the hospital. Alternative therapies may also help reduce pancreatitis pain.

You can try yoga, relaxation exercises such as deep breathing, and meditation if conventional treatments don't reduce your pain. These alternative treatments focus on slow, measured movements that can take your mind off your discomfort.

A 2017 study found that acupuncture may provide short-term pain relief for people with chronic pancreatitis. Although more studies are needed, some research has also suggested that taking antioxidant supplements may help relieve pain from pancreatitis.

Pancreatitis pain

Pain associated with pancreatitis may last from a few minutes to several hours at a time. In severe cases, discomfort from chronic pancreatitis could become constant.

Your pain is likely to increase after you eat or when you're lying down. Try sitting up or leaning forward to make yourself more comfortable.

Activities like yoga, meditation, and acupuncture may help with pain from pancreatitis. You can also try taking pain medication or antioxidant supplements to help relieve pain.

Surgery is currently a last resort for treating pancreatitis, but research from 2013 indicated that performing surgery earlier in the course of treatment may help with pain relief.

Pancreatitis complications

Some people may develop complications. These complications are rare, but they're more common in people with chronic pancreatitis:

- kidney damage

- pancreatic cancer

- diabetes

- malnutrition

- pancreatic infections

Acute pancreatitis may increase your risk of developing breathing difficulties. It can also cause pseudocysts to form when tissue and other debris collect on your pancreas. These may go away by themselves. If they rupture, it can cause infection and bleeding that can be fatal if untreated.

Pancreatitis Diet Cookbook

Vegetable Chili

Lighter than the classic beef chili, this rendition is rich in vegetables and heart health beans. Feel free to vary the beans as you like.

Serves 8

½ cup water

2 Spanish onions, coarsely chopped

4 garlic cloves, finely chopped

2 bell peppers, any combinations of colors, seeded and coarsely chopped 1 small eggplant, peeled, if desired, and cubed or 3 zucchini, cubed

1 tablespoon dried Greek oregano

1 - 2 tablespoons chili powder

2 teaspoons crushed red pepper flakes

1 tablespoon ground cumin, or more, to taste

1 teaspoon cayenne pepper (optional)

1 16 ounce can or 2 cups cooked white beans, rinsed and drained 1

16 ounce can or 2 cups cooked black beans, rinsed and drained 4 (1 pound) cans dark red kidney beans, rinsed and drained

1 cup dried lentils, washed and picked over for stones

2 20 ounce cans whole tomatoes, coarsely chopped, including juice

Freshly chopped cilantro or basil

Place the water, onions, garlic, peppers, eggplant or zucchini and spices in an 8 quart stockpot over low heat and cook until the vegetables are softened, 10-15 minutes.

Lower the heat to low, add the beans, lentils and tomatoes and cook, covered, for 1 - 2 hours, stirring occasionally. Cover and refrigerate at least overnight and up to five days. Or freeze in serving sizes up to two months.

Just prior to serving, add basil or cilantro.

Nutritional Information:

Calories 333,Total Fat 2g, Saturated Fat 0g, Trans Fat 0g, Cholesterol 0mg, Sodium 480mg, Total Carbohydrate 64g, Dietary Fiber 17g, Protein 20g

Lauren's Cauliflower Soup
Soup doesn't get simpler than this embarrassingly easy, non- fat soup. Food doesn't get plainer than this so feel free to add curry powder, a tiny bit of cream or Parmesan cheese if your diet allows, fresh basil or cilantro leaves or some Dijon mustard.

Yield: 12 cups

1 Spanish onion, chopped

5- 6 cups non-fat chicken stock

1 head cauliflower, cored and chopped

Place the onion and 2 tablespoons stock in a large saucepan over medium heat and cook until the onion gets very tender and starts to brown, about 10 minutes. Add the remaining chicken stock and bring to a boil. Lower the heat to low, cover and cook until the cauliflower is tender, about 35 minutes. Remove the solids and transfer to a food processor or blender.

Process, in batches, until smooth, gradually adding the remaining broth. Transfer to a container, cover and refrigerate up to 2 days or serve immediately.

Nutritional Information:

Calories 22,Total Fat 0g, Saturated Fat 0g, Trans Fat 0g, Cholesterol 4mg, Sodium 401mg, Total Carbohydrate 0g, Dietary Fiber 2g, Protein 1g

Carrot Soup with Ginger
Simple and inexpensive to make, silky, rich and filling, served hot or chilled, Carrot Soup with Ginger makes a great lunch, afternoon pick-me-up, or when accompanied by salad, a light dinner.

Yield: 12 cups

1 tablespoon water

1 medium Spanish onion, coarsely chopped

1 pinch ground cinnamon

1- 2 teaspoons fresh ginger root, peeled and coarsely chopped 2 pounds carrots, sliced

1 Granny Smith apple, peeled, if desired and diced 8 cups non-fat chicken stock

1/2 cup non- fat buttermilk or yogurt (optional)

Place the water, onion, cinnamon, ginger root, carrots and apple in a heavy bottomed saucepan or stockpot over medium low heat and cook until the they are beginning to soften, about 15- 20 minutes.

Add the chicken stock, raise the heat to high and bring the soup to a boil. Reduce the heat to low and cook for 30 minutes.

Transfer the soup to a blender and process until completely smooth, gradually adding the buttermilk, if desired. Serve immediately or cover and refrigerate up to 5 days.

Nutritional Information:

Calories 70,Total Fat 1g, Saturated Fat 0g, Trans Fat 0g, Cholesterol 0mg, Sodium 597mg, Total Carbohydrate 16g, Dietary Fiber 2g, Protein 5g

Lentil Barley Soup

Make this your standard lentil soup but vary the vegetables by substituting leeks or shallots for the scallions, adding zucchini or kale and replacing the barley and quinoa with brown rice for a slightly nutty flavor.

Yield: 10-12 cups

1 cup dried lentils, rinsed and picked over 4 scallions, including greens, sliced

5 carrots, chopped

3 celery stalks, including leaves, chopped

1 teaspoon dried Greek oregano

1/4 cup barley

1/4 cup quinoa, rinsed

10- 12 cups non-fat chicken or vegetable stock

1 16 ounce can diced tomatoes, including liquid Kosher

salt and black pepper to taste

1 tablespoon red wine vinegar or lemon juice

Place the lentils, scallions, carrots, celery stalks, oregano, barley, quinoa and chicken stock in a 6 quart pot and bring to a boil over a medium high heat. Reduce the heat to low and simmer, uncovered, for two hours.

Add the tomatoes and continue cooking for an additional one to two hours. Add salt and pepper to taste. Just prior to serving, add vinegar.

Nutritional Information:

Calories 96, Total Fat 1g, Saturated Fat 0g, Trans Fat 0g, Cholesterol 0mg, Sodium 160mg, Total Carbohydrate 11g, Dietary Fiber 0g, Protein 1g

Rice, potatoes and grains
Beans and Rice

Favored for its meatless high protein count, this traditional combination can be found in many different ethnic cuisines. Feel free to increase the spices, if your diet allows it.

Serves 4

2 teaspoons olive oil

2 garlic cloves, pressed or finely chopped 1 small onion, chopped

1 red bell pepper, seeded and diced

1/4 teaspoon cayenne pepper, or more to taste

1/8 teaspoon cumin, or more to taste

1 fresh or canned tomato, coarsely chopped

1 16 ounce can black beans or red kidney beans, drained and rinsed 1 -

2 cups water, non-fat chicken or vegetable stock

3 - 4 cups cooked white or brown rice Salt to taste

2 tablespoons freshly chopped cilantro (optional) or chopped Italian flat leaf parsley leaves

Place a large skillet over medium low heat and when it is hot, add the oil. Add the garlic, onion, bell pepper, cayenne and cumin and cook until the onion has softened, about 10 minutes. Reduce the heat to low, add the tomato, beans and water and cook until the beans are very soft, about 20 minutes. Add salt to taste. Serve immediately over rice and garnished with the cilantro if desired.

Nutritional Information:

Calories 302,Total Fat 3g, Saturated fat 1g, Trans Fat 0g, Cholesterol 4mg, Sodium 12mg, Total Carbohydrate 55g, Dietary Fiber 11g, Protein 13g

Overstuffed Broccoli Parmesan Potatoes
For a quick meal, roast the potatoes ahead of time and assemble just prior to eating. Feel free to substitute kale, escarole, cauliflower or broccoli rabe for the broccoli.

Serves 4

4 Idaho potatoes, pricked with a fork

1 cup non fat Greek yogurt

1/2 cup grated Parmesan cheese

2 scallions, trimmed, white and green thinly sliced

1/2 teaspoon kosher salt

1/4 teaspoon dry mustard

pinch cayenne

¼ head broccoli, lightly steamed, florets chopped, stalks peeled and finely chopped Hungarian paprika

Preheat the oven to 400 degrees.

Place the potatoes in the oven and roast until the flesh is tender and the skin is slightly hardened, about 40 minutes. Set aside for 10 minutes.

Lay the potatoes on a cutting board and cut off the uppermost ¼. Discard the top. Scoop out the flesh and place it in a medium size mixing bowl. Add the yogurt, parmesan cheese, scallions, salt, mustard and cayenne and mix until well combined. Add the broccoli and mix again. Divide into 4 portions and return the mixture to the scooped out potatoes. Sprinkle with paprika, transfer to the oven and bake until heated throughout, about 15 minutes. Serve immediately.

Nutritional Information:

Calories 373, Total Fat 4g, Saturated Fat 2g, Trans Fat 0g, Cholesterol 11mg, Sodium 236mg, Total Carbohydrate 71g, Dietary Fiber 8g, Protein 18g

Roasted Mixed Vegetables
Oven roasting is a simple, no fuss way to intensify the flavor of vegetables. It t is a method that works

well for just about every variety.

Serves 4

1 large red onion, sliced or 4 shallots1

1 red bell pepper, seeded and sliced

1 yellow squash, sliced

1 zucchini, sliced diagonally

2 cups cherry tomatoes

4 - 8 garlic cloves, in paper

1 teaspoon dried thyme, basil or rosemary

1/4 - 1/2 teaspoon kosher salt

1/4 teaspoon black

pepper 1 tablespoon olive oil

1 tablespoon balsamic vinegar

Preheat the oven to 400 degrees. Line the pan with parchment paper or a silpat.Put all the ingredients, except for the balsamic vinegar, in a baking pan and toss well.

Transfer to the oven and roast until the vegetables are browned and tender, about 1 hour. Do not crowd the pan: if necessary use two!

Transfer the vegetables to a shallow bowl and sprinkle with balsamic vinegar. Serve immediately.

Nutritional Information:

Calories 80, Total Fat 4g, Saturated Fat 1g, Trans Fat 0g, Cholesterol 0mg, Sodium 299mg, Total Carbohydrate 11g, Dietary Fiber 2g, Protein 2g

Roasted Beets with Orange and Fresh Mint
Even beet detractors will love this side dish. Roasting the beets enhances their natural sweetness and richness. Don't like mint? Simply omit it or substitute basil.

Serves 6

2 bunches beets, trimmed, greens discarded or saved for another use 2 teaspoons olive oil

3 tablespoons orange juice

4 tablespoons balsamic

vinegar 1 teaspoon Dijon

mustard

2 teaspoons finely chopped fresh mint (optional)

Kosher salt and pepper to taste

Preheat the oven to 400 degrees.

If the beets are very small, leave them whole. If they are large, quarter them and lightly rub with 1 teaspoon olive oil. Place them in a roasting pan, transfer to the oven and roast until they are soft enough to be pierced with a fork, about 1 hour.

Just prior to taking the beets out of the oven, place the orange juice, vinegar, remaining olive oil and mustard in a small pan and bring to a boil. Gently peel the beets and pour this mixture over them. Add salt and pepper to taste.

Nutritional Information:

Calories 48, Total Fat 2g, Saturated Fat 0g, Trans Fat 0g, Cholesterol 0mg, Sodium 57mg, Total Carbohydrate 7g, Dietary Fiber 1g, Protein 1g

Mashed Sweet Potatoes
So naturally rich and wonderful, you'll think you're eating dessert.

Serves 4

4 sweet potatoes, peeled, if desired and diced 2

teaspoons unsalted butter

1 tablespoon honey or maple syrup (optional)

Kosher salt, to taste

Place the potatoes in a large saucepan, cover with cold water and bring to a boil over high heat. Boil until the sweet potatoes are tender, about 20 minutes. Drain well, transfer to a bowl, add the butter and honey, if desired, and using a fork or a potato masher, mash until smooth. Add salt to taste. Serve immediately.

Nutritional Information:

Calories 153, Total Fat 3g, Saturated Fat 1g, Trans Fat 0g, Cholesterol 3mg, Sodium 73mg, Total Carbohydrate 30g, Dietary Fiber 4g, Protein 2g

Basic Risotto
A classic Northern Italian dish, risotto is creamy and comforting. This version is much lower in fat than traditional recipes.

Serves 4

1 teaspoon olive oil

1 medium Spanish onion, finely chopped 1 shallot,

finely chopped

1 1/2 cups Arborio rice (Do not substitute any other kind) 4

1/2 - 5 cups non fat chicken or vegetable stock

6 ounces baby spinach

Kosher salt and black pepper to taste

Grated Parmesan Cheese, to taste

Place a large heavy bottomed saucepan over low heat and when it is hot, add the oil. Add the onion and cook until softened, 10-15 minutes.

Add rice and sauté one minute. Add 1/2 cup stock to rice and simmer until all the stock has been absorbed, stirring constantly and slowly.

Continue adding stock until all the stock has been absorbed, continuing to add it gradually and stirring all the while.

Serve immediately, garnished with Parmesan cheese.

Nutritional Information (Cheese Included):

Calories 446, Total Fat 7g, Saturated Fat 1g, Trans Fat 0g, Cholesterol 10mg, Sodium 512mg, Total

Carbohydrate 80g, Dietary Fiber 1g, Protein 19g

Pasta
Chunky Creamy Tomato Sauce

This creamy cream-less, vegetable laden tomato sauce is wonderful on pasta, quinoa, polenta and barley.

Serves 8

1/4 cup water

2 garlic cloves, chopped

1 leek, very well washed or 1 small bunch scallions, trimmed and finely chopped 3 carrots, diced

2 tablespoons chopped fresh Italian flat leaf parsley leaves 1

28 ounce can diced tomatoes, including liquid

2 zucchini, diced

1 red bell pepper, seeded and diced

1/4 cup white wine or orange juice 1 teaspoon kosher salt

1/2 teaspoon black pepper

1/4 cup skim milk buttermilk

1/4 cup non fat Greek yogurt

1 tablespoon tomato paste

2 tablespoons chopped fresh basil leaves, plus additional for garnish 1 pound medium size shaped pasta, such as shells or rotini

Shaved or grated Parmesan cheese.

Place the water, leek, scallions, garlic, carrots, parsley, tomatoes, zucchini and red pepper in a large non stick skillet over medium high heat and cook until the vegetables begin to soften, 10-15 minutes.

Add the wine or orange juice, salt and pepper and cook until all the vegetables are soft, about 20 minutes.

Place the buttermilk, yogurt and tomato paste in a small bowl and stir to combine. Gradually add the buttermilk mixture to the skillet and cook for 2 - 3 minutes, stirring all the while. Stir in the basil.

Bring a large pot of water to a boil and cook the pasta until al dente.

Serve pasta in shallow bowls with sauce on top,

garnished with Parmesan cheese.

Nutritional Information:

Pasta Sauce Alone

Calories 52, Total Fat 0g, Saturated Fat 0g, Trans Fat 0g, Cholesterol 0mg, Sodium 464mg, Total Carbohydrate 11g, Dietary Fiber 2g, Protein 3g

Sauce with Pasta

Calories 268, Total Fat 2g, Saturated Fat 1g, Trans Fat 1g, Cholesterol 54mg, Sodium 476mg, Total Carbohydrate 51g, Dietary Fiber 3g, Protein 11g

Artichoke Tomato Sauce

Crave artichokes but don't want all the fuss? This pasta sauce includes artichoke hearts and bottoms for a rich, artichoke-y sauce. Be sure to rinse the artichokes well to get rid of any tinny flavor from the cans.

Yields about 5 - 6 cups

1 teaspoon olive oil

3- 4 garlic cloves, thinly sliced

1 small onion, thinly sliced

1 16 ounce can artichoke hearts, drained, rinsed and chopped

1 16 ounce can artichoke bottoms, drained, rinsed and chopped 1

16 ounce can diced tomatoes, including juice

1 cup water

Juice and zest of ½ lemon

¼ cup chopped fresh basil or parsley leaves

Place a large skillet over medium low heat and when it is hot, add the oil. Add the garlic and onion and cook until they are soft and golden, about 7 minutes. Raise the heat to medium high, add the artichoke hearts and cook, stirring occasionally, for five minutes. Add the tomatoes, and water and bring to a quick boil. Lower the heat to low, cover and cook 15 minutes. Add the lemon juice and zest and the basil. Serve immediately

Nutritional Information:

Calories 99, Total Fat 1g, Saturated Fat 0g, Trans Fat 0g, Cholesterol 0mg, Sodium 250mg, Total Carbohydrate 21g, Dietary Fiber 9g, Protein 6g

Pasta with Broccoli Rabe and White Beans

The combination of the bitter broccoli rabe and the creamy white beans is heavenly. If you aren't a fan of broccoli rabe, feel free to substitute broccoli or cauliflower.

Serves 4

2 teaspoons olive oil

4 garlic cloves, chopped or pressed

1 large bunch broccoli rabe, heavy stems removed and flowers coarsely chopped2 1/4 -

1/2 teaspoon crushed red pepper flakes (optional)

1 - 2 (16 ounce) cans white beans, drained and rinsed

1/2 pound medium sized, shaped pasta, such as penne, rigatoni or conchiglie

Place a large non stick skillet over medium heat and when it is hot, add the olive oil. Add the garlic and cook until just turning golden, about 2 minutes. Add the broccoli rabe, stir well and cook until the rabe begins to brighten, 3 - 5 minutes. Raise the heat to high, add red pepper flakes and white beans and cook until the beans are heated through, about 3 minutes.

Bring a large pot of water to boil. Add pasta and cook until tender. Drain pasta, reserving 1/2 cup of pasta water. Add pasta water to broccoli rabe mixture and stir to combine. Add pasta and stir. Just prior to serving, add toasted pine nuts.

Nutritional Information:

Calories 314, Total Fat 4g, Saturated Fat 1g, Trans Fat 0g, Cholesterol 0mg, Sodium 516mg, Total Carbohydrate 55g, Dietary Fiber 6g, Protein 15g

Pasta with Fresh Tomato Sauce
Dinner doesn't get any easier than this!

Serves 6

1 pound dried pasta (any shape is fine)

1 teaspoon olive oil

2 garlic cloves, thinly sliced

2 28 ounce cans plum tomatoes, drained and coarsely chopped pinch white sugar

2 - 3 tablespoons water or wine

1 tablespoon dried basil

1 teaspoon dried oregano

1/4 cup fresh chopped basil leaves

Shaved or grated Parmesan Cheese

Bring a large pot of water to boil. Add the pasta.Place a large non- stick skillet over medium heat and when it is hot, add the oil. Add the garlic and cook for 2 minutes. Add the tomatoes, sugar, water or wine, dried basil and oregano.

Cook the tomato mixture until the pasta is tender, or about 15 minutes. Drain the pasta and place equal amounts on 4 plates and top with tomato sauce. Place fresh basil on top of each bowl. Serve immediately with fresh Parmesan cheese.

Nutritional Information:

Calories 350, Total Fat 5g, Saturated Fat 1g, Trans Fat 2g, Cholesterol 73mg, Sodium 465mg, Total Carbohydrate 65g, Dietary Fiber 6g, Protein 13g

Pasta with Tomatoes and Arugula
Also known as rocket, roquette, rugula and rucola, arugula, aromatic and slightly bitter is a nice contrast to the tomatoes.

Serves 4

1 teaspoon olive oil

¼ cup chopped Prosciutto (optional)

small red onion, chopped

2 garlic cloves, minced

1 28 ounce can diced tomatoes, including the liquid

2 cups dry pasta

2 cups arugula, washed

Grated Asiago or Parmesan cheese, for serving

Place a large pot of water over high heat and bring to a boil. Add the pasta and cook according to the package instructions or until al dente, about 12 minutes. Drain, reserving ½ cup pasta water.

Place a large skillet over medium heat and add the oil. Add the onion and garlic and cook until soft, about 5 minutes. Add the tomatoes and cook 15 minutes. Add ½ cup pasta water.

Add the pasta and cook until hot, about 1- 2 minutes.

Place the arugula in the bottom of a large shallow bowl, top with the pasta mixture and toss gently. Serve immediately.

Nutritional Information:

Calories 267,Total Fat 6g, Saturated Fat 1g, Trans Fat 0g, Cholesterol 50mg, Sodium 320mg, Total Carbohydrate 46g, Dietary Fiber 2g, Protein 10g

Pasta with Broccoli, Cauliflower and Toasted Pine Nuts

A wonderful and traditional classic Italian pasta dish for those who love vegetables in the cabbage family. Roasted Brussels sprouts could be exchanged for either the broccoli or cauliflower, walnuts for the pine nuts and dried cranberries for the raisins.

Serves 4

2 teaspoons canola or olive oil

1 small Spanish onion, coarsely chopped

2 - 3 garlic cloves, finely chopped

1/2 head cauliflower, core removed, florets chopped

1/2 head broccoli, stem discarded or saved for another use, florets chopped 1 cup non fat chicken broth

1 pound medium sized, shaped pasta, such as

penne, rigatoni or conchiglie 1/4 cup pine nuts, lightly toasted

1/2 cup raisins or currants

1/2 cup grated Parmesan cheese

1/2 cup chopped fresh Italian flat leaf parsley leaves 2 tablespoons balsamic vinegar

Place a large skillet over medium heat and when it is hot, add the oil. Add the onion and garlic and cook until the onion is golden, about 10 minutes.

Add the cauliflower and broccoli florets and cook 5 minutes. Add the chicken broth and cook until the florets are almost tender, about 5 minutes.

While the sauce is cooking, place the pine-nuts, raisins, parmesan cheese, parsley and balsamic vinegar in a bowl, toss together and set aside.

Bring a large pot of water to boil. Add the pasta and cook until tender. Drain immediately and transfer to a shallow serving bowl. Add the broccoli mixture and top pine-nut mixture.

Serve immediately.

Nutritional Information:

Calories 469, Calories from Fat 177, Total Fat 14g,

Saturated Fat 3g, Trans Fat 0g, Cholesterol 93mg, Sodium 296 mg, Total Carbohydrate 110g, Dietary Fiber 7g, Protein 26g

Pasta with Roasted Bell Pepper Sauce
Roasting the bell peppers makes this sauce surprisingly delicate! Try it atop fish or chicken or even as a sandwich spread.

Serves 4

6 red, orange or yellow bell peppers

4 garlic cloves

2 tablespoons olive oil

1 pound dried pasta (any shape is fine)

1/2 cup chopped Italian flat leaf parsley or basil leaves

Parmesan cheese (optional)

Preheat broiler or oven to 500 degrees.

Place the peppers directly under the broiler, as close together as possible and broil until blackened on all sides. Place the peppers in a heavy plastic or paper bag and let sweat for about 10 minutes. Remove burned skin. Seed and stem peppers.

Place roasted peppers, garlic and olive oil in a food processor fitted with a steel blade and process until pureed.

Bring a large pot of water to a boil. Add pasta and cook until al dente. Drain pasta, reserving 1/2- 1 cup of pasta water. Add pasta water to peppers and puree. Place equal amounts of pasta in 4 bowls and top with Roasted Pepper sauce. Garnish with the parsley or basil and Parmesan, if desired.

Nutritional Information (with 1Tbsp of Cheese):

Calories 471, Calories from Fat 92, Total Fat 10g, Saturated Fat 2g, Trans Fat 0g, Cholesterol 83mg, Sodium 63mg, Total Carbohydrate 78g, Dietary Fiber 5g, Sugars 10g, Protein 16g

Pasta Fagioli
Pasta fagioli can be served as a first course, or an entree with a simple green salad and some bread.

Serves 4

1 Spanish onion, chopped

2 celery stalks, chopped

2 carrots, chopped

2 garlic cloves, finely chopped or pressed 3 cups chicken stock nonfat

1 (28 ounce) can diced tomatoes

1 teaspoon dried or 1 tablespoon chopped fresh rosemary

4 cups cooked white cannellini beans, drained and rinsed

2 cups medium sized shaped pasta, such as penne, rigatoni or conchiglie

Place a large skillet over medium low heat, add the onion, celery, carrots, garlic and ¼ cup chicken stock. Cook until the vegetables are tender, about 20 minutes.

Add the tomatoes and remaining stock. If you are using dried rosemary, add it now. Raise the heat to medium high and bring to a low boil. Reduce heat to low and cook for one hour.

Add the beans and cook until heated throughout, 5 - 10 minutes.

Bring a large pot of water to boil. Cook the pasta until al dente and transfer to a mixing bowl. Add the bean mixture and toss well. If you are using fresh rosemary, add it just prior to serving. Serve from the pot or place in a large ceramic bowl.

Nutritional Information:

Calories 395, Total Fat 5g, Saturated Fat 1g, Trans Fat 0g, Cholesterol 54mg, Sodium 607mg, Total Carbohydrate 72g, Dietary Fiber 4g, Protein 21g

Broccoli Pesto
Instead of using fresh basil leaves, this pesto is made from broccoli, for a more nutritious sauce. While it was created to use on pasta, it also makes a great addition to barley, quinoa, rice and omelets and can also be used as a dip.

Serves 4

1 small head broccoli, stems removed and saved for another use 2 garlic cloves, thinly sliced

1/3 cup grated Parmesan cheese

1 cup coarsely chopped fresh basil leaves

Fill a large bowl with cold water.

Bring a large pot of water to a boil. Add the broccoli and garlic and boil until tender, about 20 minutes. Drain and place in the bowl with cold water. Drain and transfer to food processor fitted with a steel blade. Process until totally smooth, adding Parmesan and basil at the end.

Serve immediately over just cooked pasta.

Nutritional Information:

Calories 23, Total Fat 1g, Saturated Fat 1g, Trans Fat 0g, Cholesterol 4mg, Sodium 66mg, Total Carbohydrate 1g, Dietary Fiber 0g, Protein 2g

Poultry and fish
Salmon with Mustard and Maple Syrup

A little bit of spice and a little bit of maple make this easy and quick salmon dish a perfect match for any dark green vegetable.

Serves 4

1 – 1 ¼ pound salmon filets, whole or divided into serving pieces 2 tablespoons Dijon mustard

2 tablespoons real Maple syrup

1 lemon or lime, quartered

Preheat the broiler.

Place the salmon on a baking sheet and brush with the mustard and Maple syrup. Transfer to the broiler and cook until the salmon is deeply colored, about 6 minutes. Serve immediately, garnished with the lemon.

Nutritional Information:

Calories 227, Total Fat 13g, Saturated Fat 4g, Trans Fat 0g, Cholesterol 57mg, Sodium 66mg, Total Carbohydrate 5g, Dietary Fiber 0g, Protein 23g

Salmon with Balsamic, Orange and Rosemary
If fresh rosemary isn't available, don't even think of substituting dried rosemary. Instead try fresh basil or cilantro. Serve with steamed rice, quinoa or barley and a dark green vegetable.

Serves 4

¼ cup orange juice

¼ cup balsamic vinegar

1 – 1 ¼ pounds salmon filet, whole or cut into serving pieces 1 teaspoon fresh rosemary leaves

1 tablespoon finely chopped chives

Place the orange juice and balsamic vinegar in a small pan and bring to a boil over high heat. Continue cooking until the liquid has halved, about 5 minutes. Set aside while you prepare the salmon.

To cook the salmon: Place a large non-stick pan over medium high heat and when it is hot, add the salmon. Cook until it begins to color, 3- 4 minutes on each side. Add the orange juice mixture and rosemary and cook for 1 minute. Serve immediately, garnished with the chives.

Nutritional Information:

Calories 222, Total Fat 12g, Saturated Fat 3g, Trans Fat 0g, Cholesterol 56mg, Sodium 57mg, Total Carbohydrate 4g, Dietary Fiber 0g, Protein 23g

Salmon Steaks with Herbs
These herby salmon steaks are a fantastic welcome for the spring grilling season. Try the herb paste on boneless chicken, too.

Serves 4

For the herbs:

1 tablespoons fresh basil leaves

2 tablespoons fresh cilantro leaves

¼ cup Italian flat leaf parsley leaves

2 tablespoons water

1 garlic clove

1 teaspoon dried oregano

For the salmon:

1 tablespoon olive oil

4 6-ounce salmon steaks, ¾- 1 inch thick

1 teaspoon kosher salt

½ teaspoon black pepper

To make the herb mixture: Place all the ingredients in a food processor fitted with a steel blade and process until fully chopped and as smooth as you can get it.

To cook the salmon: Place a large skillet over high heat and when it is hot, add oil. Add the salmon and cook until deeply browned, about 5 minutes on each side. Top with the herb mixture and serve immediately.

Nutritional Information:

Calories 254, Total Fat 16g, Saturated Fat 3g, Trans Fat 0g, Cholesterol 71mg, Sodium 459mg, Total Carbohydrate 1g, Dietary Fiber 0g, Protein 25g

Turkey Chili

This makes a large batch, enough for a party or enough to serve for dinner and then have leftovers for the freezer: freeze in individual containers for a quick lunch or dinner. The alcohol will cook off the beer but if you don't want to include, simply omit it. If the chili gets too thick, simply add a little bit of water.

Good accompaniments include chopped fresh basil or cilantro, chopped scallions, non- fat plain yogurt, chopped tomatoes, fresh lime quarters... the list is almost endless!

Yield: about 3 quarts

Serves 8

2 Spanish onions, finely chopped (about 4 cups)

1 red bell pepper, cut into 1/2-inch cubes

6 garlic cloves, minced

1/4 cup chili powder

1 tablespoon ground cumin

1 teaspoon crushed red pepper flakes

1 teaspoon dried Greek oregano

1/2 teaspoon

cayenne 1 bottle beer or ale

2 pounds ground turkey

2 cans (16 ounces each) black turtle beans, drained and rinsed 1

can (28 ounces) diced tomatoes, with juice

1 can (28 ounces) can tomato puree

Place a large non-stick stockpot over medium heat, add the onion, garlic, peppers, chili powder, cumin, red pepper flakes, oregano, cayenne and ¼ cup beer and cook, stirring occasionally, until all have softened but not browned, 15- 20 minutes. Add the ground turkey and cook, breaking it up with a wooden spoon, until it loses its rawness, about 5 minutes. Add the remaining beer, beans, tomatoes and tomato puree and bring to a gentle boil. Lower the heat to low and cook until the chili starts to come together, about 2 hours. Set aside to cool for 20 minutes. Transfer to a container, cover and refrigerate overnight. Reheat gently over low to medium heat.

Nutritional Information:

Calories 434, Total Fat 14g, Saturated Fat 3g, Trans Fat 0g, Cholesterol 84mg, Sodium 973mg, Total Carbohydrate 45g, Dietary Fiber 17g, Protein 34g

Dijon Pork Chops

The classic combination of mustard, apple and pork makes this dish comfort food. For even more apple, serve this with fresh applesauce.

Yield: 4

boneless pork chops, about 1 ½ pounds total

1 teaspoon kosher salt

½ teaspoon black

pepper 1 teaspoon olive

oil

3 tablespoons Dijon mustard

2/3 cup apple cider

Place a non-stick skillet over medium high heat and when it is hot, add the oil. Sprinkle the pork chops with the salt and pepper and place in the pan. Cook until lightly browned, 4- 7 minutes on each side, depending on the thickness. Transfer the chops to a platter and add the mustard and apple cider to the pan. Bring to a boil and pour over the chops. Serve immediately.

Nutritional Information:

Calories 153, Total Fat 6g, Saturated Fat 2g, Trans Fat 0g, Cholesterol 79mg, Sodium 673mg, Total Carbohydrate 2g, Dietary Fiber 0g, Sugars 2g, Protein 53g

Tuna au Poivre
Peppery, herby and lemony.

Serves 4

1 tablespoon finely grated lemon zest

3 - 4 teaspoons coarsely ground black pepper 2

garlic cloves, finely minced

2 teaspoons dried oregano

1 teaspoon kosher salt

4 6 ounce tuna

steaks 2 teaspoons

olive oil 1 lemon, quartered

Place the lemon zest, black pepper, garlic, oregano and salt on a large plate and mix to combine. Dredge both sides of the tuna in the mixture.

Place a large cast iron skillet over medium high heat and when it is hot, add the oil. Add the tuna and cook until browned, about 5 minutes on each side.

Serve immediately, garnished with the lemon quarters.

Nutritional Information:

Calories 305, Total Fat 11g, Saturated Fat 3g, Trans Fat 0g, Cholesterol 87mg, Sodium 785mg, Total Carbohydrate 4g, Dietary Fiber 1g, Protein 45g

Fish Stew
Serve this heady stew with steamed rice or French bread.

Serves 8

2 teaspoons olive oil

3 leeks, well washed, white and light green parts only, or 1 Spanish onion, chopped 2 celery stalks, diced

2 carrots, diced peeled

1 fennel bulb, tough outer layers removed, trimmed and diced 4 garlic cloves, finely chopped or pressed

1/4 teaspoon crushed red pepper

2 teaspoons dried thyme

1 bay leaf

1/4 teaspoon cayenne pepper

1/8 teaspoon crushed saffron threads

1 28 ounce can whole tomatoes, chopped, including liquid 6 cups light fish broth or non-fat chicken broth

1 cup dry white wine

Strips of zest from one orange

1 pound cod, cubed

1 pound halibut, cubed

Place a large skillet over low heat and when it is hot, add the olive oil. Add the onion, celery, carrots and fennel and cook until the onion is golden, about 10 minutes.

Add garlic, herbs and spices and cook for 5 minutes.

Add tomatoes, fish broth, wine and orange zest and cook for 20- 25 minutes.

Raise the heat to high and bring the mixture to a boil. Reduce the heat to low, add the cod and halibut and cook until the fish is starting to fall part, 10- 15 minutes.

Transfer 2 cups of the soup to a blender and process until smooth. Return to the soup. Serve immediately or cover and refrigerate up to 2 days. Serve with lemon wedges and French bread toasts or croutons.

Nutritional Information:

Calories 185, Total Fat 4g, Saturated Fat 1g, Trans Fat 0g, Cholesterol 42mg, Sodium 686mg, Total Carbohydrate 10g, Dietary Fiber 3g, Protein 27g

Grilled Salmon with Fruit and Sesame Vinaigrette
There are a ton of ingredients in this dish but after you make it once, you'll see it's well worth it.

Serves 4

4 6-ounce salmon

steaks 1 teaspoon

kosher salt

1 teaspoon black

pepper 1 teaspoon olive

oil

1 garlic clove, crushed

1 teaspoon finely chopped fresh ginger root peeled

½ cup chopped red onion

2 tablespoons sesame

seeds 1/4 cup lemon or lime juice

¼ cup orange, apple or pineapple juice

¼ teaspoon white sugar

1 tablespoon balsamic vinegar

1 tablespoon finely chopped fresh basil or cilantro leaves 2 scallion greens, finely chopped

¼- ½ teaspoon kosher salt

Prepare the grill or preheat the broiler.

Sprinkle the salmon with the salt and pepper. When the grill is hot, place the steaks on the grill and cook 5- 6 minutes on each side. Alternatively, place under the broiler.

In the meantime, place a large skillet over medium heat and when it is hot, add the oil. Add the garlic, ginger root, onion and sesame seeds and cook until the vegetables are soft and the seeds are lightly browned, about 5 minutes. Off heat, add the juices, sugar, vinegar, basil or cilantro, scallion greens, salt and pepper.

When the steaks are ready, top with the vinaigrette. Serve immediately.

Nutritional Information:

Calories 380, Calories from Fat 207, Total Fat 23g, Saturated Fat 23g, Trans Fat 0g, Cholesterol 84mg, Sodium 373mg, Total Carbohydrate 7g, Dietary Fiber 1g, Sugars 3g,

Protein 35g

Roasted Chicken

If you know how to cook only one thing, this is it. Feel free to add hard vegetables like potatoes, onions, shallots, carrots, sweet potatoes, turnips, beets and butternut squash to the pan while you roast the chicken. You can also stuff the cavities with fresh rosemary, thyme or parsley leaves and/or lemon, apple or onions, or a combination.

Serves 6

1 whole roaster chicken, about 6 - 7 pounds

1 - 1 1/2 teaspoons kosher salt

1/4 teaspoon black pepper

Preheat oven to 450 degrees. Remove and discard giblets and neck from chicken cavity. Rinse chicken in several changes of cold water and pat dry.

Rub skin and flesh with kosher salt and black pepper. Place on roasting rack in pan. Transfer to oven and roast the juices run clear from the breast and the leg moves easily and the internal temperature is about 160 degrees, about 70 minutes (10 minutes per pound).

Do not baste. Cut the chicken into serving pieces and remove the skin.

Nutritional Information:

Calories 235, Total Fat 6g, Saturated Fat 2g, Trans Fat 0g, Cholesterol 128mg, Sodium 539mg, Total Carbohydrate 0g, Dietary Fiber 0g, Protein 42g

Turkey Meatloaf

This lighter meatloaf is great for dinner but equally delicious leftover in a sandwich. Serves 10

1 teaspoon olive oil

1 small Spanish onion, chopped

2 - 3 garlic cloves, finely chopped or pressed

1 teaspoon dried Greek oregano

2 - 3 tablespoons Dijon mustard

1/2 teaspoon black pepper

1/4 - 1/2 teaspoon salt

3/4 cup tomato ketchup or barbecue sauce

1/2 cup chopped fresh Italian flat leaf parsley leaves

2 slices good quality white bread

1/2 cup beef or chicken stock none fat

1 large egg, lightly beaten

2 pounds lean ground chicken or turkey

Preheat the oven to 350 degrees. Lightly grease an 8 x 4 inch loaf pan.

Place a medium size skillet over low heat and when it is hot, add the oil. Add the onion, garlic and oregano and cook until the onion is golden, about 10 minutes. Transfer to a large mixing bowl and set aside to cool. In the meantime, soak the bread in the stock until it is moist, about 2 minutes. Drain off as much liquid as possible. Add the bread to the cooled onion mixture.

Add the eggs and ground meat and mix, by hand , until everything is thoroughly incorporated. Place the mixture in the prepared loaf pan, transfer to the oven and cook for about 1 hour and 15 minutes.

Nutritional Information:

Calories 162, Total Fat 8g, Saturated Fat 2g, Trans Fat 0g, Cholesterol 61mg, Sodium 397mg,

Total Carbohydrate 8g, Dietary Fiber 0g, Protein 14g

Basic Burger with Toppings
Whether made with ground beef, turkey, chicken, lamb or pork, there are endless ways to eat a burger.

6 ounces low-fat ground turkey or chicken, formed into a patty

Kosher salt and pepper

1. Preheat broiler. Sprinkle with salt and pepper. Place patty on a broiler pan or baking sheet about 2 1/2- 3 inches from the broiler and broil for about 5 minutes perside.

OR......

2. Sprinkle with salt and pepper. Heat a large cast iron skillet and when droplets of water bounce off, add the hamburger patty. Cook for about 5 minutes on each side.

OR........

3. Prepare grill. Sprinkle with salt and pepper. Place burger on grill and cook for about 5 minutes on each side.

WHEN THE BURGER IS COOKED, ADD (but just remember the additions change the nutritional information):

Lettuce

Tomatoes

Ketchup

Relish

Raw red onions, soaked in boiling water for 5 minutes

Guacamole

Salsa

Caramelized onions

Roasted peppers

Roasted garlic

Mustard

Chili sauce

Barbecue sauce

Nutritional Information:

Calories 183, Total Fat 2g, Saturated Fat 0g, Cholesterol 106mg, Sodium 84mg, Total Carbohydrate 0g, Dietary Fiber 0g

Vietnamese Style Chicken

Steamed green beans and brown rice complete this to make a great weekday dinner.

Serves 4

2 tablespoons plus 1/3 cup water

¼ cup Asian fish sauce

2 large shallots or 1 small onion, finely chopped 2 garlic cloves, minced

Pinch black pepper

Pinch crushed red pepper flakes

¼ cup sugar

1 ½ pounds boneless skinless chicken breasts (2 large), each breast half cut in half

¼ cup chopped fresh basil or cilantro leaves

Place the 2 tablespoons water and Asian fish sauce in a small bowl and set aside. Place the shallots, garlic, black and red peppers in another small bowl and set aside.

Place the remaining 1/3 cup water and the sugar in a large skillet and cook over medium heat until the sugar has caramelized into a deep brown, about 6 minutes.

Remove the pan from the heat, and .very carefully (to avoid splattering) add the fish sauce mixture to the pan. Return to the heat and cook until the mixture boils. 1-2 minutes. Add the shallot mixture and cook until the shallots have softened, about 3 minutes. Add the chicken, in a single layer, and cook, stirring occasionally, until cooked throughout, about

4 minutes per side. Serve immediately, sprinkled with the basil.

Nutritional Information:

Calories 374, Total Fat 8g, Saturated Fat 2g, Trans Fat 3g, Cholesterol 155mg, Sodium 1526mg, Total Carbohydrate 15g, Dietary Fiber 0g, Protein 58g

Pan Grilled Chicken with Lemon and Basil

Serve with steamed brown or white rice and a chopped tomato salad.

Serves 4

1 ½ pounds boneless, skinless chicken breasts, pounded thin and sliced lengthwise to get 4 cutlets

¼ cup fresh lemon juice

¼ cup chopped fresh basil leaves

1 teaspoon dried oregano

½ teaspoon black pepper

½ teaspoon kosher salt

Place the chicken, lemon juice, basil and oregano in a non-reactive glass or ceramic bowl and mix to combine. Cover and refrigerate at least 2 but no more than 4 hours.

Drain the chicken and discard the marinade. Sprinkle with the salt and pepper.Place a large cast iron skillet over medium high heat and when it is almost smoking hot, add the chicken, waiting for the pan to reheat between additions. Cook until golden brown, just firm to the touch and cooked throughout, about 4 minutes per side, depending on the thickness of the chicken.

Nutritional Information:

Calories 324,Total Fat 8g, Saturated Fat 2g, Trans Fat 03g, Cholesterol 155mg, Sodium 430mg, Total Carbohydrate 3g, Dietary Fiber 0g, Protein 57g

Desserts
Grilled Pineapple

A superb dessert to make when you already have the grill going, this low-calorie, low- fat treat is easy and impressive.

Serves 4

1 tablespoon unsalted butter

2 teaspoons brown sugar

Juice of ½ lime

1 fresh pineapple, cored and cut into eighths, lengthwise

Place the butter, brown sugar and lime juice in a small bowl and mix well.

Prepare a grill or preheat the broiler.

Brush butter mixture on the pineapple, place on the grill or under the broiler and cook, turning once, until lightly browned on both sides, about 4 minutes. Drizzle with the remaining butter mixture.

Nutritional Information:

Calories 142, Total Fat 3g, Saturated Fat 1g, Trans Fat 0g, Cholesterol 3mg, Sodium 4mg,

Total Carbohydrate 21g, Dietary Fiber 3g, Protein 1g

9 798665 042091